A Natural Approach to Cure Diabetes

Revitalize Your Well-being Through Natural Solutions

JAMES BRANDY

INTRODUCTION

Welcome to "Reclaiming Health: A Natural Approach to Diabetes Cure." In this comprehensive guide, we begin on a journey toward understanding and overcoming diabetes through natural means.

Diabetes, a chronic condition affecting millions worldwide, is characterized by high blood sugar levels. Its prevalence continues to rise, necessitating a deeper understanding of its types, symptoms, and underlying causes.

In this introductory chapter, we lay the foundation for our exploration. We delve into the intricacies of diabetes, examining its various types, ranging from type 1, an autoimmune condition, to type 2, often associated with lifestyle factors. We discuss the telltale signs and symptoms, empowering readers to recognize potential indicators and seek timely intervention.

Moreover, we emphasize the pivotal role of lifestyle in managing diabetes. While medical interventions are essential, the choices we make in our daily lives profoundly influence our health outcomes. From dietary habits to physical activity levels, each aspect plays a crucial role in diabetes prevention and management.

As we embark on this journey together, let us embrace a holistic approach to health—one that honors the interconnectedness of mind, body, and spirit. By reclaiming our health through natural means, we can unlock the potential for healing and vitality.

CHAPTER ONE

The Foundations of Natural Healing

In our quest to reclaim health and combat diabetes naturally, it is essential to understand the foundational principles of holistic healing. This chapter serves as a cornerstone for our journey, exploring the interconnectedness of mind, body, and spirit, as well as the guiding principles of natural medicine and healing.

Exploring Holistic Health: Mind, Body, and Spirit

Holistic health is rooted in the understanding that the mind, body, and spirit are intricately interconnected, influencing one another in profound ways. Rather than treating symptoms in isolation, holistic healing acknowledges the whole person, considering all aspects of their being.

The mind-body connection underscores the profound impact of mental and emotional well-being on physical health. Stress, anxiety, and unresolved emotions can manifest as physical ailments, exacerbating conditions such as diabetes. By nurturing mental and emotional wellness through mindfulness, stress management techniques, and emotional healing practices, we can promote overall health and vitality.

Moreover, holistic health recognizes the importance of spiritual well-being in fostering resilience and inner peace. Cultivating a sense of purpose, connection to something greater than oneself, and engaging in practices such as meditation and prayer can nourish the spirit and enhance overall well-being.

Principles of Natural Medicine and Healing

Natural medicine embraces the innate healing capacity of the body and seeks to support and enhance its self-healing mechanisms. At its core, natural medicine is guided by several fundamental principles:

The Healing Power of Nature: Nature provides a wealth of healing resources, from medicinal herbs and plants to fresh air and sunlight. Natural medicine harnesses the therapeutic properties of nature to promote health and well-being.

Identify and Treat the Root Cause: Rather than merely addressing symptoms, natural medicine aims to identify and address the underlying root cause of illness or imbalance. By treating the root cause, true healing can occur, leading to long-lasting results.

Do No Harm: Natural medicine prioritizes gentle, non-invasive therapies that support the body's innate healing processes without causing harm or adverse side effects.

Treat the Whole Person: Natural medicine considers the individual as a whole, taking into account their physical, mental, emotional, and spiritual dimensions. Treatment plans are personalized to address the unique needs of each individual.

By embracing these principles and adopting a holistic approach to health and healing, we lay the groundwork for reclaiming our health and achieving optimal well-being. In the chapters that follow, we will delve deeper into specific strategies and practices for combating diabetes naturally, guided by these foundational principles of natural healing.

Nutrition plays a pivotal role in managing and reversing diabetes naturally. In this chapter, we explore the transformative power of plant-based eating, delve into the concepts of glycemic index and glycemic load, and highlight essential nutrients for diabetes management.

The Power of Plant-Based Eating

Plant-based eating has emerged as a cornerstone of diabetes management and reversal, offering a wealth of health benefits. A plant-based diet focuses on whole, minimally processed foods derived from plants, including fruits, vegetables, legumes, whole grains, nuts, and seeds. Embracing a predominantly plant-based diet can significantly improve blood sugar control, reduce insulin resistance, and lower the risk of diabetes-related complications.

The abundance of fiber found in plant-based foods plays a crucial role in diabetes management. Fiber helps slow the absorption of sugar into the bloodstream, preventing spikes in blood sugar levels and promoting greater insulin sensitivity. Additionally, plant-based diets are rich in antioxidants, vitamins, and minerals, which support overall health and reduce inflammation—a key factor in diabetes progression.

Understanding Glycemic Index and Glycemic Load

The concepts of glycemic index (GI) and glycemic load (GL) are invaluable tools for understanding how different foods affect blood sugar levels. The glycemic index measures how quickly a carbohydrate-containing food raises blood sugar levels compared to pure glucose, which has a GI of 100. Foods with a high GI cause rapid spikes in blood sugar, while those with a low GI result in slower, more progressive increases.

Glycemic load takes into account both the quality and quantity of carbohydrates in a serving of food, providing a more comprehensive picture of its impact on blood sugar levels. While some foods may have a high glycemic index, their glycemic load may be low if they contain relatively small amounts of carbohydrates per serving.

By choosing foods with a low glycemic index and glycemic load, individuals with diabetes can better manage their blood sugar levels and reduce the risk of complications.

Essential Nutrients for Diabetes Management

In addition to paying attention to carbohydrate quality and quantity, individuals with diabetes should focus on incorporating essential nutrients that support blood sugar control and overall health. Key nutrients for diabetes management include:

Omega-3 fatty acids: Found in fatty fish, flaxseeds, chia seeds, and walnuts, omega-3 fatty acids help reduce inflammation and improve insulin sensitivity.

Magnesium: Magnesium plays an important role in glucose metabolism and insulin action. Notable dietary sources include leafy green vegetables, nuts, seeds, and whole grains.

Chromium: Chromium enhances the action of insulin and helps regulate blood sugar levels. It can be found in broccoli, barley, oats, and green beans.

Vitamin D: Adequate vitamin D levels are associated with improved insulin sensitivity and reduced risk of type 2 diabetes. Food sources include fatty fish, fortified dairy products, and sunlight exposure.

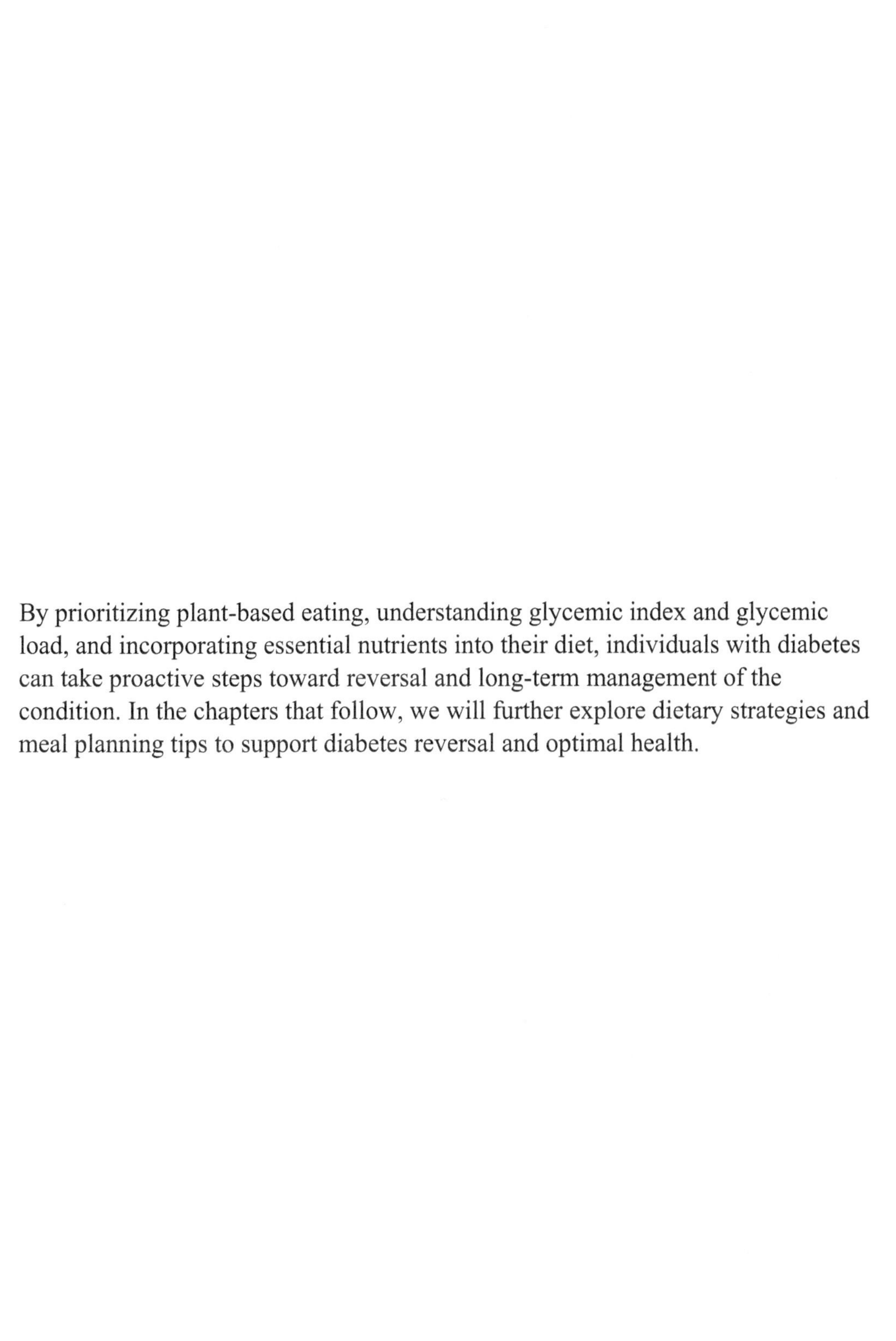

By prioritizing plant-based eating, understanding glycemic index and glycemic load, and incorporating essential nutrients into their diet, individuals with diabetes can take proactive steps toward reversal and long-term management of the condition. In the chapters that follow, we will further explore dietary strategies and meal planning tips to support diabetes reversal and optimal health.

Herbal remedies and supplements offer natural alternatives to conventional medications for managing diabetes and promoting overall health. In this chapter, we delve into the therapeutic properties of herbs and highlight key supplements that can help balance blood sugar levels.

Harnessing the Healing Properties of Herbs

For centuries, herbs have been used in traditional medicine systems worldwide for their medicinal properties. Many herbs possess anti-diabetic effects, helping to improve insulin sensitivity, reduce blood sugar levels, and protect against diabetes-related complications.

1. Cinnamon: Cinnamon is renowned for its ability to improve insulin sensitivity and lower blood sugar levels. It contains compounds that mimic the action of insulin, facilitating glucose uptake by cells. Incorporating cinnamon into our diet, either through supplementation or spicing it into foods and beverages, can help regulate blood sugar levels.

2. Ginseng: Ginseng is an adaptogenic herb known for its ability to enhance overall health and vitality. Several studies have shown that ginseng may improve insulin sensitivity, lower fasting blood sugar levels, and reduce postprandial glucose spikes. It can be consumed as a tea, in supplement form, or added to recipes.

3. Fenugreek: Fenugreek seeds are rich in soluble fiber, which helps slow down the absorption of carbohydrates and stabilize blood sugar levels. Fenugreek supplementation has been shown to improve glycemic control and reduce insulin resistance in individuals with diabetes.

4. Bitter melon: Bitter melon, also known as bitter gourd, contains compounds that mimic the action of insulin and help regulate blood sugar levels. Consuming bitter melon extract or juice may help improve glucose tolerance and insulin sensitivity.

5. Berberine: Berberine is a plant compound found in several herbs, including goldenseal, Oregon grape, and barberry. It has been extensively studied for its anti-diabetic properties, with research suggesting that it can lower blood sugar levels, improve insulin sensitivity, and reduce inflammation.

Key Supplements for Balancing Blood Sugar Levels

In addition to herbal remedies, certain supplements can play a beneficial role in managing diabetes and supporting overall health. These supplements are often used as adjunctive therapies to conventional treatment regimens:

1. Alpha-lipoic acid: Alpha-lipoic acid is a powerful antioxidant that helps reduce oxidative stress and improve insulin sensitivity. It has been shown to decrease fasting blood sugar levels and improve symptoms of diabetic neuropathy.

2. Chromium: Chromium is an essential mineral that plays an important role in glucose metabolism. Supplementing with chromium picolinate or chromium polynicotinate may help improve insulin sensitivity and regulate blood sugar levels.

3. Magnesium: Magnesium deficiency is common in individuals with diabetes and has been associated with insulin resistance and poor glycemic control. Supplementing with magnesium may help improve insulin sensitivity and lower the risk of diabetes-related complications.

4. Omega-3 fatty acids: Omega-3 fatty acids, found in fish oil supplements, flaxseed oil, and algae oil, have anti-inflammatory properties and may help improve insulin sensitivity. Incorporating omega-3 supplements into your diet can support overall cardiovascular health and reduce the risk of diabetes-related complications.

Before incorporating herbal remedies or supplements into your diabetes management plan, it is essential to consult with a healthcare provider, especially if you are taking medications or have underlying health conditions. By harnessing the healing properties of herbs and integrating key supplements into your routine, you can take proactive steps toward balancing blood sugar levels and promoting optimal health and well-being.

Physical activity and exercise are integral components of diabetes management, offering numerous benefits for controlling blood sugar levels and improving overall health. In this chapter, we explore the importance of tailoring exercise to manage diabetes effectively and highlight the various benefits of regular physical activity for diabetes control.

Tailoring Exercise to Manage Diabetes

When it comes to managing diabetes through exercise, one size does not fit all. The key is to tailor exercise regimens to individual needs, taking into account factors such as age, fitness level, mobility, and any existing health conditions. By working closely with healthcare providers and exercise professionals, individuals with diabetes can develop personalized exercise plans that are safe, effective, and enjoyable.

1. Cardiovascular Exercise: Cardiovascular exercise, such as walking, jogging, swimming, cycling, or dancing, is essential for improving cardiovascular health, increasing endurance, and burning calories. Aerobic activities help lower blood sugar levels by raising insulin sensitivity and promoting muscle glucose uptake.

2. Strength Training: Strength training, also known as resistance or weight training, involves using weights, resistance bands, or bodyweight exercises to build and strengthen muscles. Strength training can help improve insulin sensitivity, increase muscle mass, and enhance metabolic function, leading to better blood sugar control over time.

3. Flexibility and Balance Exercises: Flexibility and balance exercises, such as yoga, tai chi, and Pilates, can help improve range of motion, reduce stiffness, and

enhance balance and coordination. These exercises are particularly beneficial for individuals with diabetes who may experience neuropathy or other complications affecting mobility and flexibility.

4. Interval Training: Interval training involves alternating between high-intensity bursts of activity and periods of rest or low-intensity exercise. This form of exercise can be especially effective for individuals with diabetes, as it helps improve cardiovascular fitness, burn calories, and enhance insulin sensitivity in a shorter amount of time.

Benefits of Consistent Physical Activity for Diabetes Control

Regular physical activity offers a multitude of benefits for individuals with diabetes, including:

Improved Blood Sugar Control: Physical activity helps lower blood sugar levels by increasing insulin sensitivity and promoting glucose uptake by muscles.

Weight Management: Exercise plays a crucial role in weight management by burning calories and promoting fat loss, which can help reduce insulin resistance and improve blood sugar control.

Reduced Risk of Complications: Regular physical activity can help reduce the risk of diabetes-related complications, such as heart disease, stroke, neuropathy, and kidney disease.

Enhanced Cardiovascular Health: Exercise strengthens the heart and blood vessels, lowers blood pressure and cholesterol levels, and improves overall cardiovascular function, reducing the risk of heart disease and stroke.

Improved Mood and Well-being: Physical activity releases endorphins, neurotransmitters that promote feelings of happiness and well-being, and helps reduce stress, anxiety, and depression often associated with diabetes.

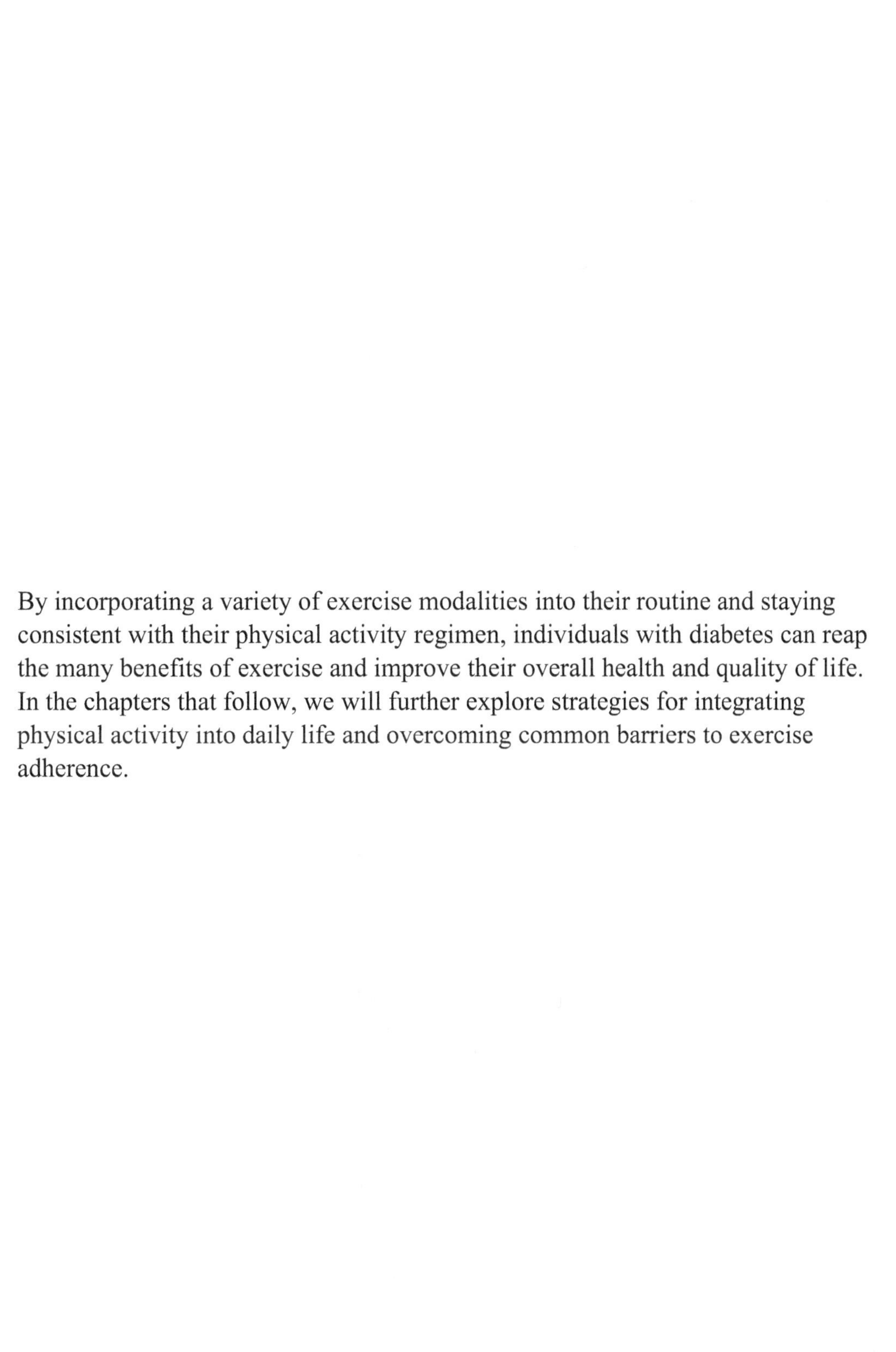

By incorporating a variety of exercise modalities into their routine and staying consistent with their physical activity regimen, individuals with diabetes can reap the many benefits of exercise and improve their overall health and quality of life. In the chapters that follow, we will further explore strategies for integrating physical activity into daily life and overcoming common barriers to exercise adherence.

CHAPTER FIVE

Stress Management and Mind-Body Practices

Stress has a profound impact on both our physical and mental well-being, including its influence on blood sugar levels. In this chapter, we explore the relationship between stress and diabetes, and we delve into mindfulness, meditation, and relaxation techniques as effective tools for managing stress and promoting overall health.

Stress and How It Influences Blood Sugar Levels

When we experience stress, whether it's from work, relationships, financial worries, or other life challenges, our bodies respond by releasing stress hormones such as cortisol and adrenaline. These hormones trigger the "fight or flight" response, preparing the body to respond to perceived threats. While this response can be life-saving in acute situations, chronic stress can have detrimental effects on our health, including our blood sugar levels.

Stress-induced spikes in cortisol and adrenaline can cause blood sugar levels to rise temporarily. This is because these hormones stimulate the liver to release glucose into the bloodstream, providing energy to cope with the perceived threat. For individuals with diabetes, whose bodies may already struggle to regulate blood sugar levels, chronic stress can exacerbate the problem, leading to difficulty in managing diabetes and increased risk of complications.

Moreover, stress can also impact behaviors related to diabetes management, such as overeating, unhealthy food choices, lack of physical activity, and medication non-adherence. These behaviors can further contribute to blood sugar imbalances and worsen diabetes control over time.

Mindfulness, Meditation, and Relaxation Techniques

Fortunately, there are effective strategies for managing stress and mitigating its impact on blood sugar levels. Mind-body practices such as mindfulness, meditation, and relaxation techniques offer powerful tools for cultivating inner peace, reducing stress, and promoting overall well-being.

1. Mindfulness: Mindfulness involves paying attention to the present moment with openness, curiosity, and acceptance. By cultivating mindfulness, we can become more aware of our thoughts, feelings, and bodily sensations, allowing us to respond to stressors more skillfully and reduce their impact on our health.

2. Meditation entails instructing the mind to nurture tranquility, clarity, and concentration. Through various meditation techniques, such as mindfulness meditation, loving-kindness meditation, and body scan meditation, we can quiet the chatter of the mind, reduce stress, and promote relaxation.

CHAPTER SIX

Lifestyle Adjustments for Long-Term Success

In our quest to reclaim health and achieve long-term success in managing diabetes, lifestyle adjustments play a crucial role. In this chapter, we explore how to create a supportive environment for healthier living and discuss strategies for overcoming challenges and staying motivated on the journey toward optimal well-being.

Creating a Supportive Environment for Healthier Living

Our environment plays a significant role in driving our behaviors and habits. By creating a supportive environment that fosters healthier living, we can set ourselves up for success in managing diabetes and achieving our wellness goals.

1. Healthy Eating Environment: Stocking our kitchens with nutritious foods and minimizing the presence of unhealthy, processed snacks can make it easier to make healthier food choices. Surrounding ourselves with fruits, vegetables, whole grains, and lean proteins encourages us to nourish our bodies with wholesome, diabetes-friendly meals.

2. Physical Activity Integration: Incorporating physical activity into our daily routines can be facilitated by creating an environment that supports movement. This may involve setting up a home gym or designating a space for exercise, scheduling regular walks or bike rides, and choosing active leisure activities that we enjoy.

3. Social Support Network: Surrounding ourselves with supportive friends, family members, or support groups can provide encouragement, accountability, and motivation on our wellness journey. Engaging in activities with like-minded individuals who share similar health goals can make it easier to stay on track and overcome challenges together.

4. Stress Reduction Techniques: Cultivating a stress-free environment can help reduce the likelihood of stress-related blood sugar spikes. This may involve creating a calming atmosphere at home, practicing relaxation techniques such as deep breathing or meditation, and setting boundaries to protect our mental and emotional well-being.

Overcoming Challenges and Staying Motivated

While embarking on a journey toward healthier living, it's essential to anticipate and address potential challenges that may arise along the way. By adopting a proactive mindset and implementing strategies to stay motivated, we can navigate obstacles and maintain momentum toward our wellness goals.

1. Goal Setting: Setting specific, measurable, achievable, relevant, and time-bound (SMART) goals can provide clarity and direction on our wellness journey. Breaking larger goals into smaller, manageable steps can make them more attainable and increase our sense of accomplishment along the way.

2. Tracking Progress: Monitoring our progress, whether it's tracking food intake, physical activity, blood sugar levels, or other health metrics, can help us stay accountable and identify areas for improvement. Using tools such as food journals, activity trackers, or diabetes management apps can make tracking progress convenient and accessible.

3. Celebrate Achievements: Celebrating milestones and achievements, no matter how small, can boost our confidence and motivation to continue making progress. Rewarding ourselves for reaching goals with non-food rewards, such as treating ourselves to a relaxing massage or enjoying a favorite hobby, reinforces positive behaviors and fosters a sense of accomplishment.

4. Seeking Support: Don't hesitate to reach out for support from healthcare providers, diabetes educators, or trusted loved ones when facing challenges or feeling discouraged. Seeking guidance, encouragement, and practical tips from others who understand our journey can provide invaluable support and motivation to persevere.

By creating a supportive environment for healthier living, anticipating and addressing challenges, and staying motivated through goal setting, progress tracking, celebrating achievements, and seeking support, we can lay the foundation for long-term success in managing diabetes and reclaiming our health. In the chapters that follow, we will further explore strategies for sustainable lifestyle adjustments and overcoming common barriers to wellness.

CHAPTER SEVEN

Success Stories and Real-Life Transformations

In this chapter, we shine a spotlight on inspiring accounts of individuals who have successfully reversed diabetes naturally through lifestyle changes, dietary modifications, and holistic approaches to health. These real-life transformations serve as a source of inspiration and motivation for others embarking on their journey toward reclaiming health and wellness.

1. Mary's Story: Mary was diagnosed with type 2 diabetes and struggled for years to manage her blood sugar levels with medications. Frustrated by the side effects and lack of progress, she decided to take control of her health through lifestyle changes. By adopting a plant-based diet, incorporating regular exercise into her routine, and practicing stress reduction techniques, Mary was able to reverse her diabetes and achieve optimal health.

2. Stanley's Journey: Stanley, a busy professional with a sedentary lifestyle, was shocked when he received a diagnosis of prediabetes. Determined to avoid developing full-blown diabetes, he committed to making healthier choices. With the support of a nutritionist and personal trainer, Stanley revamped his diet, started exercising regularly, and prioritized stress management. Within months, his blood sugar levels returned to normal, and he regained his vitality and energy.

3. Ruth's Triumph: Ruth struggled with type 1 diabetes for years, relying on insulin injections to manage her condition. Despite her challenges, she refused to let diabetes define her. Through diligent research and experimentation, Ruth discovered the power of holistic healing modalities, including herbal remedies, acupuncture, and energy healing. With the guidance of integrative healthcare practitioners, Ruth was able to reduce her dependence on insulin and achieve greater stability in her blood sugar levels.

4. John's Path to Wellness: John was diagnosed with gestational diabetes during his wife's pregnancy, prompting him to reevaluate his lifestyle choices. Concerned about his long-term health and the impact of diabetes on his family, John committed to making lasting changes. He embraced a low-carbohydrate, whole-food diet, engaging in regular physical activity, and practiced mindfulness to manage stress. Consequently, John not only successfully reversed his prediabetes but also motivated his entire family to embrace healthier lifestyles.

These success stories highlight the transformative power of lifestyle interventions and holistic approaches to diabetes management. By taking proactive steps to reclaim their health, these individuals not only reversed their diabetes but also experienced profound improvements in their overall well-being. Their journeys serve as a testament to the potential for positive change and offer hope to others seeking to overcome diabetes naturally.

In the chapters that follow, we will continue to explore practical strategies, evidence-based approaches, and expert insights to support individuals on their path to wellness. Whether you're newly diagnosed with diabetes or looking to optimize your health, these real-life transformations demonstrate that with dedication, determination, and support, reclaiming health is within reach.

2. Tracking Progress: Monitoring our progress, whether it's tracking food intake, physical activity, blood sugar levels, or other health metrics, can help us stay accountable and identify areas for improvement. Using tools such as food journals, activity trackers, or diabetes management apps can make tracking progress convenient and accessible.

3. Celebrate Achievements: Celebrating milestones and achievements, no matter how small, can boost our confidence and motivation to continue making progress. Rewarding ourselves for reaching goals with non-food rewards, such as treating ourselves to a relaxing massage or enjoying a favorite hobby, reinforces positive behaviors and fosters a sense of accomplishment.

4. Seeking Support: Don't hesitate to reach out for support from healthcare providers, diabetes educators, or trusted loved ones when facing challenges or

feeling discouraged. Seeking guidance, encouragement, and practical tips from others who understand our journey can provide invaluable support and motivation to persevere.

By creating a supportive environment for healthier living, anticipating and addressing challenges, and staying motivated through goal setting, progress tracking, celebrating achievements, and seeking support, we can lay the foundation for long-term success in managing diabetes and reclaiming our health. In the chapters that follow, we will further explore strategies for sustainable lifestyle adjustments and overcoming common barriers to wellness.

CHAPTER EIGHT

Family and Community Support

In the journey to manage diabetes and embrace natural healing, the support of family and community can make a significant difference. This chapter explores the importance of building a supportive network for diabetes management and the value of educating loved ones about diabetes and natural healing.

Building a Supportive Network for Diabetes Management

1. Open Communication: Communication is key in fostering a supportive environment for diabetes management. Encourage open and honest conversations with family members, friends, and healthcare providers about your diabetes diagnosis, treatment plan, and wellness goals. Sharing your experiences, concerns, and needs can help others understand how they can best support you on your journey.

2. Team Approach: Diabetes management is a team effort that involves not only the individual with diabetes but also their family members, caregivers, and healthcare professionals. Collaborate with your support network to develop a comprehensive care plan that addresses your physical, emotional, and social needs. Regularly involve family members in medical appointments, discussions about treatment options, and decisions regarding lifestyle changes.

3. Emotional Support: Living with diabetes can be emotionally challenging, and having a supportive network can provide invaluable emotional support. Lean on your loved ones for encouragement, empathy, and reassurance during difficult times. Joining support groups or online communities for individuals with diabetes and their families can also provide a sense of belonging and camaraderie.

Educating Loved Ones About Diabetes and Natural Healing

1. Understanding Diabetes: Educate your family members about diabetes, including its causes, symptoms, treatment options, and potential complications. Provide resources such as books, articles, and reputable websites to help them gain a better understanding of the condition and its impact on your life.

2. Promoting Healthy Lifestyle Choices: Encourage your loved ones to join you in making healthier lifestyle choices that support diabetes management and overall well-being. Involve them in meal planning, grocery shopping, and physical activities that promote nutritious eating and regular exercise. Emphasize the importance of stress management, adequate sleep, and other lifestyle factors in diabetes prevention and management.

3. Exploring Natural Healing: Educate your family members about the principles of natural healing and the role of lifestyle interventions, dietary modifications, and holistic approaches in diabetes management. Share success stories and real-life examples of individuals who have reversed diabetes naturally, highlighting the transformative power of lifestyle changes and integrative therapies.

By building a supportive network for diabetes management and educating loved ones about diabetes and natural healing, you can create an environment that fosters understanding, empathy, and collaboration. Together, you can navigate the challenges of diabetes with greater resilience, unity, and hope. In the chapters that follow, we will continue to explore practical strategies, evidence-based approaches, and expert insights to support you and your support network on your journey to wellness.

CHAPTER NINE

Integrating Traditional and Modern Medicine

In the pursuit of managing diabetes and embracing natural healing, it's essential to recognize the complementary roles of traditional and modern medicine. This chapter explores the importance of understanding the role of conventional treatments and bridging the gap between natural approaches and medical care.

Understanding the Role of Conventional Treatments

Conventional treatments for diabetes typically include medications, insulin therapy, and medical interventions aimed at controlling blood sugar levels and preventing complications. While these treatments are essential for managing the condition, they may come with side effects and limitations. It's crucial to understand the role of conventional treatments and their potential benefits and drawbacks.

1. Medications: Oral medications such as metformin, sulfonylureas, and DPP-4 inhibitors are commonly prescribed to lower blood sugar levels and improve insulin sensitivity in individuals with type 2 diabetes. Insulin therapy may be necessary for individuals with type 1 diabetes or advanced type 2 diabetes who require additional support in managing blood sugar levels.

2. Monitoring: Regular monitoring of blood sugar levels, A1C levels, blood pressure, cholesterol levels, and other relevant biomarkers is essential for assessing diabetes control and adjusting treatment regimens as needed. Continuous glucose monitoring (CGM) devices and insulin pumps can provide real-time data and support more precise diabetes management.

3. Medical Interventions: In some cases, medical interventions such as angioplasty, bypass surgery, or amputation may be necessary to address complications

associated with diabetes, such as cardiovascular disease, peripheral neuropathy, or diabetic foot ulcers. These interventions aim to improve quality of life and prevent further complications.

Bridging the Gap Between Natural Approaches and Medical Care

While conventional treatments are vital for managing diabetes, natural approaches can complement medical care by addressing underlying factors contributing to the condition and promoting overall health and wellness. Bridging the gap between natural approaches and medical care involves integrating evidence-based strategies from both modalities to create a comprehensive and personalized treatment plan.

1. Holistic Assessment: A holistic assessment considers the individual as a whole, taking into account physical, mental, emotional, and spiritual aspects of health. By collaborating with healthcare providers who embrace a holistic approach, individuals with diabetes can receive personalized care that addresses their unique needs and preferences.

2. Lifestyle Modifications: Lifestyle modifications, including dietary changes, regular physical activity, stress management techniques, and adequate sleep, play a central role in diabetes management and prevention. Integrating natural approaches such as plant-based eating, herbal remedies, and mind-body practices can support conventional treatments and enhance overall well-being.

3. Shared Decision-Making: Shared decision-making involves active collaboration between individuals with diabetes and their healthcare providers in making informed decisions about treatment options and goals of care. By fostering open communication, mutual respect, and trust, individuals can actively participate in their healthcare decisions and advocate for their preferences and values.

4. Continued Monitoring and Evaluation: Regular monitoring and evaluation of diabetes control, treatment outcomes, and overall health status are essential for assessing the effectiveness of integrated treatment approaches. Adjustments to treatment regimens can be made based on individual responses, preferences, and goals.

By integrating traditional and modern medicine, individuals with diabetes can access the full spectrum of treatment options and achieve optimal outcomes in managing their condition. By embracing a collaborative and holistic approach to diabetes care, we can bridge the gap between natural approaches and medical care, empowering individuals to reclaim their health and well-being. In the chapters that follow, we will further explore practical strategies, evidence-based approaches, and expert insights to support integrated diabetes management and holistic wellness.

Monitoring and tracking progress are essential components of effective diabetes management, allowing individuals to assess their health status, track changes over time, and make informed decisions about treatment and lifestyle adjustments. In this chapter, we explore how to implement effective self-monitoring techniques and leverage technology for diabetes management and tracking.

Implementing Effective Self-Monitoring Techniques

Self-monitoring techniques enable individuals with diabetes to monitor key indicators of their health and well-being, including blood sugar levels, dietary intake, physical activity, medication adherence, and overall health status. By regularly monitoring these parameters, individuals can identify trends, detect patterns, and make informed decisions to optimize their diabetes management.

1. Blood Sugar Monitoring: Regular monitoring of blood sugar levels is crucial for individuals with diabetes to assess their glycemic control and make adjustments to their treatment regimens as needed. Self-monitoring of blood glucose (SMBG) involves using a blood glucose meter to measure blood sugar levels at various times throughout the day, such as before and after meals, before bedtime, and during periods of physical activity.

2. Food and Beverage Tracking: Keeping track of dietary intake can help individuals with diabetes make more informed food choices, monitor carbohydrate intake, and maintain overall nutritional balance. Food journals, smartphone apps, or online tracking tools can be used to record meals, snacks, portion sizes, and nutrient content, allowing for better self-awareness and accountability.

3. Physical Activity Tracking: Keeping tabs on physical activity can assist individuals managing diabetes in monitoring their exercise routines, establishing fitness objectives, and evaluating their advancements over time. Pedometers, fitness trackers, or smartphone applications with activity monitoring capabilities can furnish immediate insights into steps taken, distance covered, calories expended, and exercise duration.

4. Medication Adherence: Adhering to medication regimens is essential for managing diabetes and preventing complications. Using medication reminders, pill organizers, or smartphone apps can help individuals stay organized and compliant with their prescribed treatment plans.

Using Technology for Diabetes Management and Tracking

Technological advancements have transformed the landscape of diabetes management, providing cutting-edge tools and devices to simplify monitoring, enhance precision, and increase convenience. Through the utilization of technology, individuals with diabetes can obtain instantaneous data, acquire insights into their health condition, and make better-informed choices regarding their healthcare.

1. Continuous Glucose Monitoring (CGM) Systems: CGM systems use wearable sensors to continuously measure glucose levels in the interstitial fluid, providing real-time data on blood sugar trends, patterns, and fluctuations. CGM systems can help individuals with diabetes make timely adjustments to their insulin dosing, dietary intake, and physical activity levels to optimize glycemic control.

2. Insulin Pumps: Insulin pumps deliver insulin continuously or in predetermined doses throughout the day, mimicking the function of a healthy pancreas. Integrated with CGM technology, insulin pumps can automatically adjust insulin delivery based on real-time glucose readings, reducing the risk of hypo- and hyperglycemia.

3. Smartphone Apps and Digital Health Platforms: Smartphone apps and digital health platforms offer a wide range of features and functionalities to support diabetes management and tracking. These apps may include tools for blood sugar monitoring, food and activity tracking, medication reminders, virtual coaching, and data analysis, empowering individuals to take a proactive role in their care.

4. Telemedicine and Remote Monitoring: Telemedicine and remote monitoring technologies enable individuals with diabetes to connect with healthcare providers virtually, receive personalized guidance and support, and access remote monitoring services for ongoing management and follow-up care.

By implementing effective self-monitoring techniques and leveraging technology for diabetes management and tracking, individuals with diabetes can take a proactive approach to their care, optimize their treatment outcomes, and achieve greater control over their health and well-being. In the chapters that follow, we will further explore practical strategies, evidence-based approaches, and expert insights to support effective monitoring, tracking, and management of diabetes.

CHAPTER ELEVEN

Sustainable Habits for Lifelong Health

Creating sustainable habits is essential for achieving lasting results in diabetes management and overall health and wellness. In this chapter, we explore strategies for creating sustainable routines and preventing diabetes relapse while maintaining progress over the long term.

Creating Sustainable Routines for Lasting Results

1. Consistency over Perfection: Focus on consistency rather than perfection when establishing healthy habits. Aim for small, manageable changes that you can maintain over time, rather than drastic overhauls that may be difficult to sustain. Consistent habits, even if they seem small, can lead to significant improvements in health and well-being over the long term.

2. Gradual Progression: Gradually introduce new habits into your routine to avoid overwhelm and increase the likelihood of success. Start with one or two changes at a time, such as incorporating more fruits and vegetables into your diet or adding a short daily walk to your schedule. As these habits become ingrained, gradually add more changes to build upon your progress.

3. Mindful Eating: Practice mindful eating by paying attention to hunger and fullness cues, savoring each bite, and eating slowly. Avoid distractions such as television or screens while eating, and tune in to your body's signals to prevent overeating and promote a healthy relationship with food.

4. Regular Physical Activity: Make physical activity a regular part of your routine by scheduling regular workouts or activities that you enjoy. Aim for a mix of aerobic exercise, strength training, and flexibility exercises to support overall

health and fitness. Find activities that you look forward to and that fit into your lifestyle to increase the likelihood of sticking with them over the long term.

Strategies for Preventing Diabetes Relapse and Maintaining Progress

1. Self-Reflection and Evaluation: Regularly reflect on your progress, identify areas for improvement, and evaluate which strategies are working well for you. Adjust your approach as needed to address challenges and maintain motivation.

2. Setting Realistic Goals: Set realistic, achievable goals that align with your values and priorities. Break larger goals into smaller, manageable steps, and celebrate each milestone along the way to maintain motivation and momentum.

3. Building a Support Network: Surround yourself with supportive friends, family members, or support groups who can provide encouragement, accountability, and motivation. Share your goals and progress with others, and enlist their support in helping you stay on track.

4. Seeking Professional Guidance: Don't hesitate to seek guidance from healthcare providers, diabetes educators, or other professionals who can provide expert advice and support. Regular check-ins with your healthcare team can help you stay on track and address any challenges or concerns that arise.

By incorporating sustainable habits into your daily routine and implementing strategies to prevent diabetes relapse, you can achieve lasting results in diabetes management and overall health and wellness. With commitment, consistency, and support, you can reclaim your health and enjoy a fulfilling, vibrant life free from the limitations of diabetes. In the chapters that follow, we will continue to explore practical strategies, evidence-based approaches, and expert insights to support your journey toward lifelong health and well-being.

CHAPTER TWELVE

Celebrating Your Health Journey

In this chapter, we take a moment to reflect on personal achievements and milestones in your health journey. We explore the importance of cultivating gratitude and a positive outlook for continued wellness.

Reflecting on Personal Achievements and Milestones

1. Recognize Progress: Set aside moments to recognize and rejoice in the advancements you've achieved on your health journey. Reflect upon the beneficial alterations you've instituted, regardless of their magnitude, and acknowledge the endeavors you've undertaken to enhance your health and overall well-being.

2. Celebrate Milestones: Celebrate milestones and achievements along the way, whether it's reaching a weight loss goal, improving blood sugar control, or adopting a new healthy habit. Celebrating these accomplishments reinforces positive behavior and motivates you to continue moving forward.

3. Embrace setbacks as opportunities for learning: Acknowledge that setbacks and obstacles are inherent components of any health journey. Rather than allowing them to dishearten you, perceive setbacks as chances for personal development and education. Extract valuable lessons from setbacks and utilize them to guide future choices and behaviors.

4. Cultivate self-compassion: Extend kindness and self-compassion to yourself as you navigate the highs and lows of your health journey. Treat yourself with the same level of understanding and empathy that you would extend to a friend confronting similar challenges.

Cultivating Gratitude and Positive Outlook for Continued Wellness

1. Focus on Gratitude: Cultivate an attitude of gratitude by focusing on the positive aspects of your life and health. Take time each day to reflect on the things you're grateful for, whether it's supportive relationships, moments of joy, or improvements in your health.

2. Stay Present: Practice mindfulness and stay present in the moment, appreciating the beauty and richness of life as it unfolds. By staying present, you can fully experience the joys and blessings that surround you, enhancing your overall sense of well-being.

3. Visualize Your Future Self: Visualize your future self living a vibrant, healthy life, free from the limitations of diabetes. Use visualization techniques to imagine yourself achieving your health goals and living your best life, filled with energy, vitality, and joy.

4. Surround Yourself with Positivity: Surround yourself with positivity and uplifting influences, whether it's supportive friends and family members, inspirational books and podcasts, or uplifting affirmations and mantras. Choose to focus on what brings you joy and empowers you to thrive.

By celebrating your health journey, acknowledging personal achievements and milestones, and cultivating gratitude and a positive outlook, you can continue to nurture your well-being and thrive on your path to lifelong health and wellness. In the chapters that follow, we will continue to explore practical strategies, evidence-based approaches, and expert insights to support your ongoing journey toward optimal health and vitality.

Celebrating Your Health Journey

Your health journey is a remarkable and personal voyage filled with triumphs, challenges, and moments of growth. In this chapter, we take a moment to reflect on your achievements and milestones and explore the power of cultivating gratitude and maintaining a positive outlook for continued wellness.

Reflecting on Personal Achievements and Milestones

1. Acknowledge Progress: Take a moment to acknowledge and celebrate the progress you've made on your health journey. Whether it's making healthier food choices, achieving weight loss goals, or improving your fitness levels, each step forward is a significant achievement worth celebrating.

2. Celebrate Milestones: Celebrate the milestones along your health journey, both big and small. Whether it's reaching a certain blood sugar level, reducing medication dosages, or incorporating regular physical activity into your routine, these milestones represent your dedication and perseverance.

3. Embrace Setbacks as Learning Opportunities: Setbacks are a natural part of any journey, including your health journey. Instead of viewing setbacks as failures, embrace them as valuable learning opportunities. Reflect on what you've learned from setbacks and use them to fuel your growth and resilience.

4. Practice Self-Compassion: Treat yourself with gentleness and practice self-compassion when faced with adversity. Understand that you are giving your best with the resources and understanding available to you, and extend kindness and empathy to yourself, particularly in moments of hardship.

Cultivating Gratitude and Positive Outlook for Continued Wellness

1. Focus on Gratitude: Cultivate an attitude of gratitude by focusing on the positive aspects of your health and life. Take time each day to reflect on the things you're grateful for, whether it's the support of loved ones, moments of joy and laughter, or the opportunity to prioritize your health.

2. Remain in the Present: Cultivate mindfulness and remain fully present in each moment, embracing the beauty and depth of life as it unfolds. By staying grounded in the present, you can immerse yourself in the abundance of blessings and possibilities that exist, enriching your overall state of well-being.

3. Visualize Your Future Self: Envision your future self to live a vibrant, healthy life filled with vitality and purpose. Use visualization techniques to imagine yourself achieving your health goals, overcoming obstacles, and embracing each day with renewed energy and enthusiasm.

4. Surround Yourself with Positivity: Encircle yourself with uplifting influences that inspire and uplift you. Surround yourself with supportive friends and family members, participate in activities that bring you happiness and satisfaction, and prioritize focusing on what enables you to flourish on your path to better health.

By reflecting on your achievements and milestones, cultivating gratitude, and maintaining a positive outlook, you can continue to nurture your well-being and thrive on your path to lifelong health and wellness. In the chapters that follow, we will continue to explore practical strategies, evidence-based approaches, and expert insights to support your ongoing journey toward optimal health and vitality.

Embracing Conclusion:

In the journey of reclaiming health and embracing a natural approach to diabetes cure, we have embarked on a transformative voyage filled with insight, empowerment, and hope. From understanding the foundations of natural healing to integrating traditional and modern medicine, each chapter has been a stepping stone toward reclaiming control over our health and well-being.

Throughout this book, we have explored the power of lifestyle interventions, dietary modifications, and holistic approaches in managing diabetes and promoting overall wellness. We have learned how to harness the healing properties of herbs, embrace the benefits of physical activity, and cultivate resilience through stress management and mind-body practices.

We have celebrated the stories of individuals who have reclaimed their health and reversed diabetes naturally, serving as beacons of inspiration and motivation for others on their healing journey. We have reflected on personal achievements, cultivated gratitude, and maintained a positive outlook for continued wellness.

As we conclude this book, let us remember that the journey to reclaiming health is not a destination but a lifelong commitment—a journey of self-discovery, growth, and empowerment. It is about embracing a mindset of possibility, resilience, and self-compassion as we navigate the twists and turns of our health journey.

Regardless of your position on the journey to wellness, always bear in mind that you are not solitary. You are backed by a community of individuals who share your goals and obstacles, and who are present to encourage and motivate you throughout your endeavors.

As you continue on your journey, may you embrace each day with renewed determination, courage, and grace. May you honor your body, mind, and spirit with kindness and compassion, and may you reclaim your health and vitality with unwavering resolve.

With dedication, perseverance, and the belief in the power of natural healing, you have the opportunity to rewrite your health story and reclaim the vibrant, fulfilling life you deserve. Embrace this moment, embrace this journey, and embrace the limitless potential within you to reclaim your health and thrive.

Thank you for joining me on this transformative odyssey of reclaiming health. May your path be illuminated with health, happiness, and boundless vitality. Here's to your continued wellness and the extraordinary journey that lies ahead.